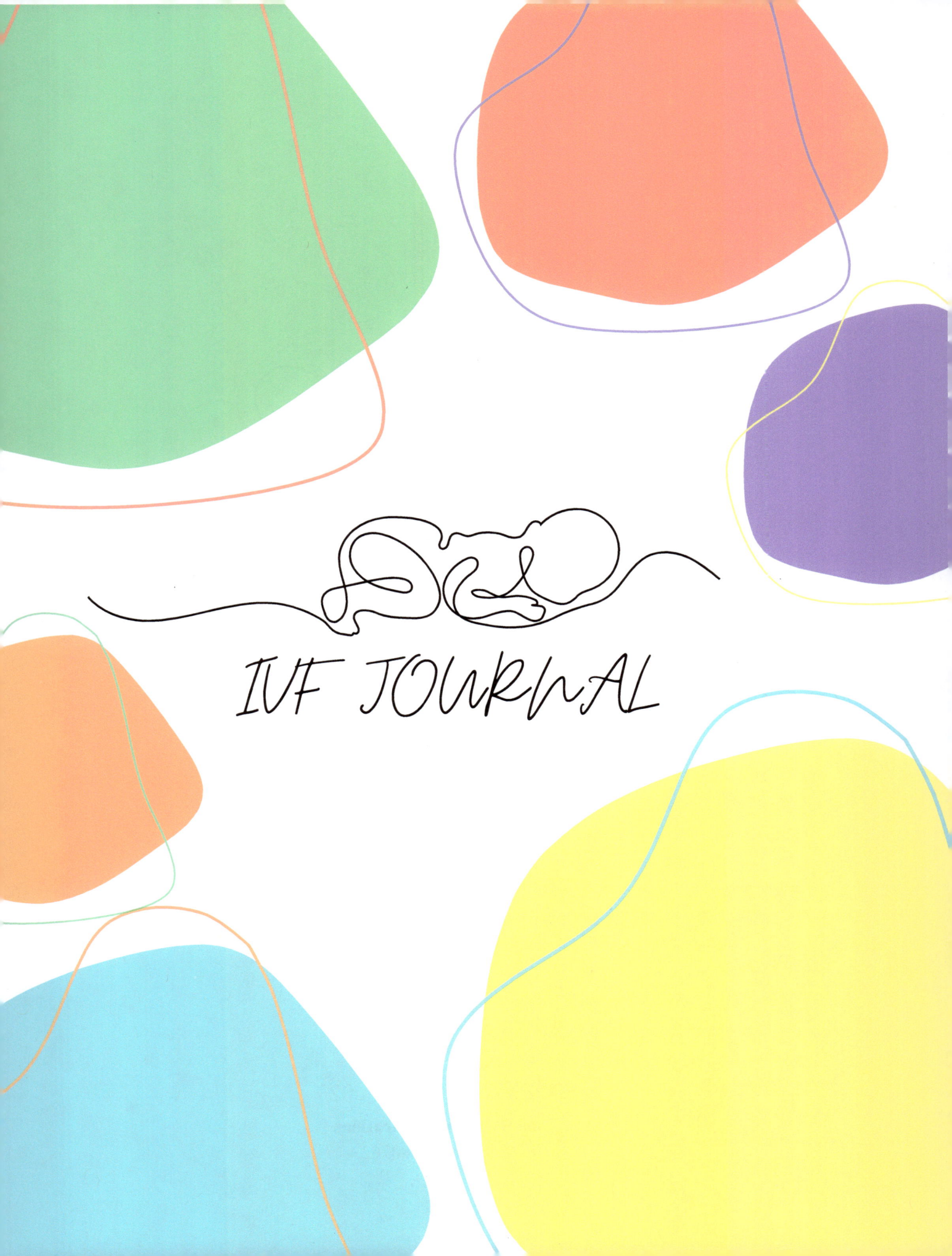

IVF JOURNAL
by Kylie Bragdon

COPYRIGHT © 2023
Line By Lions Publications
ISBN: 9781948807623

Dedicated to anyone who ever needed help being hopeful.
~Kylie

This journal belongs to...

Table of Contents

- Introduction: Your story, current concerns, potential challenges, supports, ways of practicing self-care.

- Biology: Egg and Sperm

- Appointments and Medications

- Trimester One: Size, Major milestones, and moments to remember

- Trimester Two: Size, Major milestones, and moments to remember.

- Trimester: Size, Major milestones, and moment to remember.

- Final Planning: Baby shower, baby names, and birthing plan.

INTRODUCTION

I am beginning this journey today because...

The story, up until this moment...

My current concerns about the process include...

_____
_____
_____
_____
_____
_____
_____
_____
_____

I anticipate the following challenges...

_____
_____
_____
_____
_____
_____
_____
_____
_____

During this process, my supports will include...

_____
_____
_____
_____
_____
_____
_____
_____

🔴 🟠 🟡 🟢 🔵 🔵 🟣

I will practice self-care in the following ways...

_____
_____
_____
_____
_____
_____
_____
_____

BIOLOGY

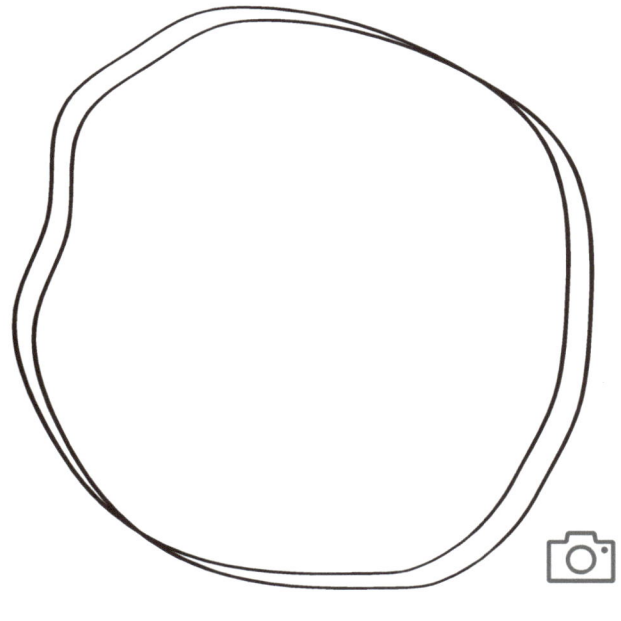

Hobbies/Interests

Characteristics

Height
Hair Color
Eye Color
Skin Tone
Body Type
Face Shape
Facial Features
Hand Size
Foot Size
Dominate Hand

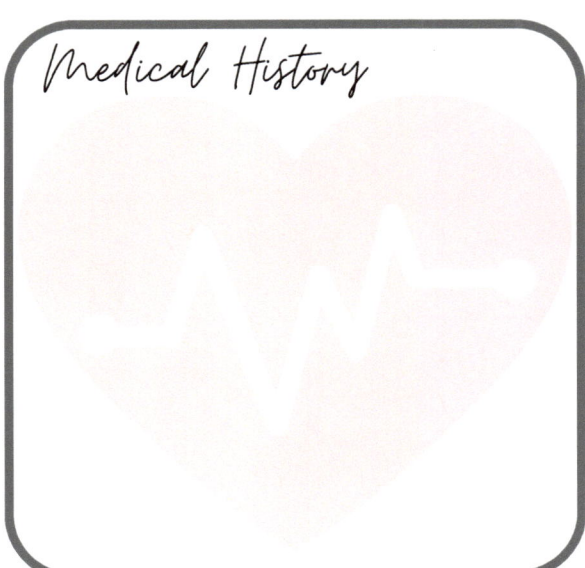

Medical History

Fun Fact

Personality Traits

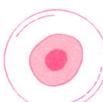

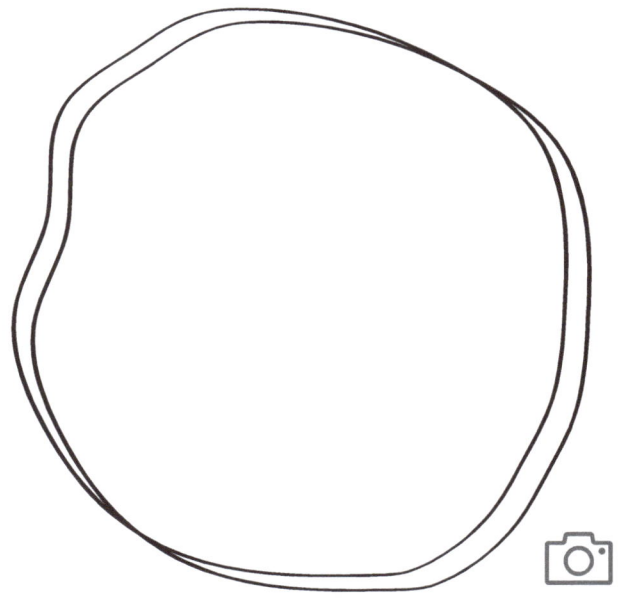

Hobbies/Interests

Characteristics

Height
Hair Color
Eye Color
Skin Tone
Body Type
Face Shape
Facial Features
Hand Size
Foot Size
Dominate Hand

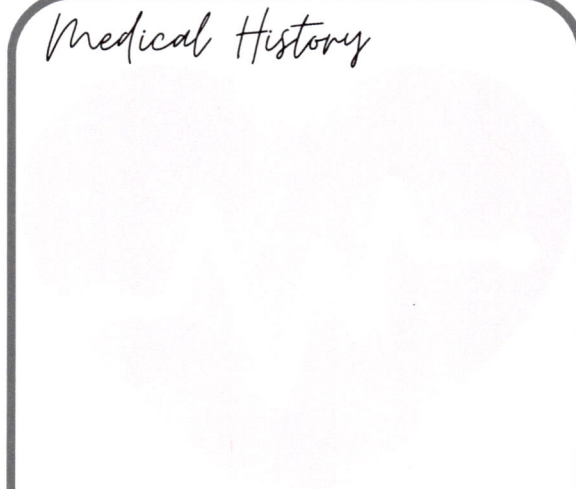

Medical History

Fun Fact

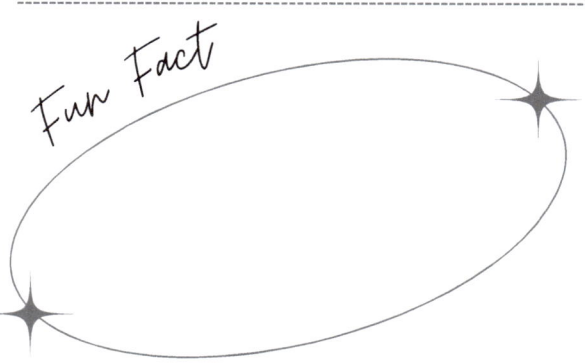

Personality Traits

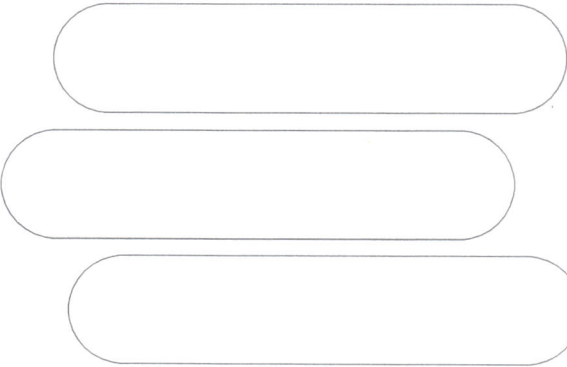

Hobbies/Interests

-
-
-
-

Characteristics

Height: ....
Hair Color: ....
Eye Color: ....
Skin Tone: ....
Body Type: ....
Face Shape: ....
Facial Features: ....
Hand Size: ....
Foot Size: ....
Dominate Hand: ....

Medical History

Personality Traits

-
-
-

Fun Fact

Characteristics

Height
_____

Hair Color
_____

Eye Color
_____

Skin Tone
_____

Body Type
_____

Face Shape
_____

Facial Features
_____

Hand Size
_____

Foot Size
_____

Dominate Hand
_____

Fun Fact

4 Hobbies/Interests

Medical History

3 Personality Traits

APPOINTMENTS

Cycle Calendar

Month _____

S	M	T	W	TH	F	S

Key Dates

-
-
-
-

Cycle Calendar

Month _____

S	M	T	W	TH	F	S

Key Dates

-
-
-
-

Appointment

Doctor: _____ Date: _____

Purpose of Appointment: _____

Questions

- [ ] 1 _____
  _____
- [ ] 2 _____
  _____
- [ ] 3 _____
  _____
- [ ] 4 _____
  _____
- [ ] 5 _____
  _____
- [ ] 6 _____
  _____
- [ ] 7 _____
  _____
- [ ] 8 _____
  _____

Notes

1 _____
  _____
2 _____
  _____
3 _____
  _____
4 _____
  _____
5 _____
  _____
6 _____
  _____
7 _____
  _____
8 _____
  _____

"Hope is the thing with feathers that perches in the soul and sings the tune without the words and never stops at all."
—Emily Dickinson

Next Steps: _____

_____

Appointment

Provider_____ Date_____

Purpose of Appointment:_____

Questions

1 _____
_____
2 _____
_____
3 _____
_____
4 _____
_____
5 _____
_____
6 _____
_____
7 _____
_____
8 _____
_____

Notes

1 _____
_____
2 _____
_____
3 _____
_____
4 _____
_____
5 _____
_____
6 _____
_____
7 _____
_____
8 _____
_____

"Pregnancy the genesis of miracles."
-Unknown

Next Steps:_____
_____

Appointment

Provider _____ Date _____

Purpose of Appointment _____

Questions

- [ ] 1 _____
      _____
- [ ] 2 _____
      _____
- [ ] 3 _____
      _____
- [ ] 4 _____
      _____
- [ ] 5 _____
      _____
- [ ] 6 _____
      _____
- [ ] 7 _____
      _____
- [ ] 8 _____
      _____

Notes

1 _____
  _____
2 _____
  _____
3 _____
  _____
4 _____
  _____
5 _____
  _____
6 _____
  _____
7 _____
  _____
8 _____
  _____

"Every journey begins with a single step. Embrace the unknown, for it is on the path of discovery that we find ourselves"
— Maya Angelou

Next Steps _____
_____

Appointment

Provider_____ Date_____

Purpose of Appointment:_____

Questions

☐ 1_____
_____

☐ 2_____
_____

☐ 3_____
_____

☐ 4_____
_____

☐ 5_____
_____

☐ 6_____
_____

☐ 7_____
_____

☐ 8_____
_____

Notes

1_____
_____

2_____
_____

3_____
_____

4_____
_____

5_____
_____

6_____
_____

7_____
_____

8_____
_____

"Hope fuels the soul's ascent."
-Unknown

Next Steps:_____
_____

Appointment

Provider_____ Date_____

Purpose of Appointment_____

Questions

- [ ] 1_____
     _____
- [ ] 2_____
     _____
- [ ] 3_____
     _____
- [ ] 4_____
     _____
- [ ] 5_____
     _____
- [ ] 6_____
     _____
- [ ] 7_____
     _____
- [ ] 8_____
     _____

Notes

1_____
_____
2_____
_____
3_____
_____
4_____
_____
5_____
_____
6_____
_____
7_____
_____
8_____
_____

"Every journey, no matter how challenging, holds the promise of transformation and personal growth."
-Oprah Winfrey

Next Steps_____

_____

Appointment

Provider_____ Date_____

Purpose of Appointment_____

Questions

1. _____
   _____
2. _____
   _____
3. _____
   _____
4. _____
   _____
5. _____
   _____
6. _____
   _____
7. _____
   _____
8. _____
   _____

Notes

1. _____
   _____
2. _____
   _____
3. _____
   _____
4. _____
   _____
5. _____
   _____
6. _____
   _____
7. _____
   _____
8. _____
   _____

"Hope is the heartbeat of resilience"
—Brene Brown

Next Steps_____

_____

Appointment

Provider_____ Date_____

Purpose of Appointment_____

Questions	Notes
☐ 1_____	1_____
☐ 2_____	2_____
☐ 3_____	3_____
☐ 4_____	4_____
☐ 5_____	5_____
☐ 6_____	6_____
☐ 7_____	7_____
☐ 8_____	8_____

"Journeys are the stories we write with our footsteps"
-Glennon Doyle

Next Steps_____

_____

Appointment

Provider_____ Date_____

Purpose of Appointment:_____

Questions

1 _____
_____
2 _____
_____
3 _____
_____
4 _____
_____
5 _____
_____
6 _____
_____
7 _____
_____
8 _____
_____

Notes

1 _____
_____
2 _____
_____
3 _____
_____
4 _____
_____
5 _____
_____
6 _____
_____
7 _____
_____
8 _____
_____

"Pregnancy is the ultimate act of faith in the beauty of creation."
— Serena Williams

Next Steps:_____
_____

Appointment

Provider_____ Date_____

Purpose of Appointment_____

Questions

☐ 1_____

☐ 2_____

☐ 3_____

☐ 4_____

☐ 5_____

☐ 6_____

☐ 7_____

☐ 8_____

Notes

1_____

2_____

3_____

4_____

5_____

6_____

7_____

8_____

"the most precious jewels you'll ever have around your neck are the arms of your children."
-Diana, Princess of Wales

Next Steps_____

_____

Appointment

Provider_____ Date_____

Purpose of Appointment:_____

Questions

1 _____
_____
2 _____
_____
3 _____
_____
4 _____
_____
5 _____
_____
6 _____
_____
7 _____
_____
8 _____
_____

Notes

1 _____
_____
2 _____
_____
3 _____
_____
4 _____
_____
5 _____
_____
6 _____
_____
7 _____
_____
8 _____
_____

"Motherhood is a journey of selflessness, where every sacrifice is a testament to unconditional love."
-Beyoncé

Next Steps:_____
_____

Appointment

Provider_____ Date_____

Purpose of Appointment_____

Questions

- [ ] 1_____
     _____
- [ ] 2_____
     _____
- [ ] 3_____
     _____
- [ ] 4_____
     _____
- [ ] 5_____
     _____
- [ ] 6_____
     _____
- [ ] 7_____
     _____
- [ ] 8_____
     _____

Notes

1_____
_____
2_____
_____
3_____
_____
4_____
_____
5_____
_____
6_____
_____
7_____
_____
8_____
_____

"the greater the obstacle, the more glorious the triumph."
-Amelia Earhart

Next Steps_____
_____

Appointment

Provider _____ Date _____

Purpose of Appointment: _____

Questions

1 _____
_____
2 _____
_____
3 _____
_____
4 _____
_____
5 _____
_____
6 _____
_____
7 _____
_____
8 _____
_____

Notes

1 _____
_____
2 _____
_____
3 _____
_____
4 _____
_____
5 _____
_____
6 _____
_____
7 _____
_____
8 _____
_____

"happiness is not determined by what we have, but by how we embrace and appreciate what we have."
-Jennifer Aniston

Next Steps _____
_____

Appointment

Provider_____ Date_____

Purpose of Appointment_____

Questions

- [ ] 1_____
  _____
- [ ] 2_____
  _____
- [ ] 3_____
  _____
- [ ] 4_____
  _____
- [ ] 5_____
  _____
- [ ] 6_____
  _____
- [ ] 7_____
  _____
- [ ] 8_____
  _____

Notes

1_____
_____
2_____
_____
3_____
_____
4_____
_____
5_____
_____
6_____
_____
7_____
_____
8_____
_____

"Hope is the heartbeat of resilience. It whispers, 'You can. You will. Keep Going.'"
~Simone Biles

Next Steps_____
_____

Appointment

Provider _____   Date _____

Purpose of Appointment _____

Questions

1 _____
_____
2 _____
_____
3 _____
_____
4 _____
_____
5 _____
_____
6 _____
_____
7 _____
_____
8 _____
_____

Notes

1 _____
_____
2 _____
_____
3 _____
_____
4 _____
_____
5 _____
_____
6 _____
_____
7 _____
_____
8 _____
_____

"The future belongs to those who believe in the beauty of their dreams."
— Eleanor Roosevelt

Next Steps _____

_____

Appointment

Provider_____ Date_____

Purpose of Appointment:_____

Questions

- [ ] 1_____
      _____
- [ ] 2_____
      _____
- [ ] 3_____
      _____
- [ ] 4_____
      _____
- [ ] 5_____
      _____
- [ ] 6_____
      _____
- [ ] 7_____
      _____
- [ ] 8_____
      _____

Notes

1_____
_____
2_____
_____
3_____
_____
4_____
_____
5_____
_____
6_____
_____
7_____
_____
8_____
_____

"family is the anchor that grounds us, the shelter that embraces us, and the love that nourishes our souls"
-Angelina Jolie

Next Steps:_____
_____

Medication log

Date/Time	Medication/Amount	Injection site	Mood

Medication log

Date/Time	Medication/Amount	Injection Site	Mood

Medication log

Date/Time	Medication/Amount	Injection Site	Mood

Medication log

Date/Time	Medication/Amount	Injection Site	Mood

Medication log

Date/Time	Medication/Amout	Injection Site	Mood

Medication log

Date/Time	Medication/Amount	Injection Site	Mood

Egg Retrieval

Date

Time

Location

Procedure Performed By

Feelings and Reflection

_____
_____
_____
_____
_____
_____

Things to Remember

-
-

Embryo Transfer

Date

Time

Location

Procedure Performed By

Feelings and Reflection

_____
_____
_____
_____
_____

Things to Remember

-
-

Pregnancy Test

Date

Time

Location

Results

Feelings and Reflection

_____
_____
_____
_____
_____

Things to Remember

-
-

Embryo Transfer

Date

Time

Location

Procedure Performed By

Feelings and Reflection

_____
_____
_____
_____
_____

Things to Remember

-
-

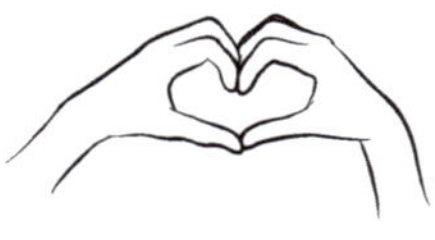

Pregnancy Test

Date

Time

Location

Results

Feelings and Reflection

_____
_____
_____
_____
_____
_____

Things to Remember

-
-

Embryo Transfer

Date

Time

Location

Procedure Performed By

Feelings and Reflection

_____
_____
_____
_____
_____

Things to Remember

-
-

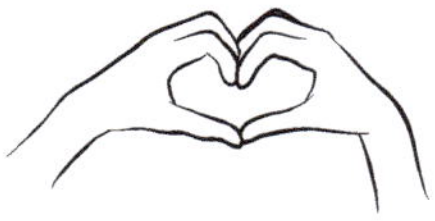

Pregnancy Test

Date

Time

Location

Results

Feelings and Reflection

_____
_____
_____
_____
_____

Things to Remember

-
-

FIRST TRIMESTER

Week 4

Baby's Size

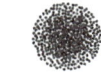

Poppy Seed

Major Milestones

- implantation occurs
- increased levels of the pregnancy hormone hCG
- the embryo begins to experience rapid cell developments

Symptoms

Cravings

Mood Meter
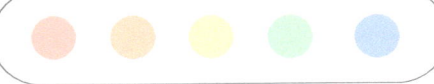

Sleep Meter
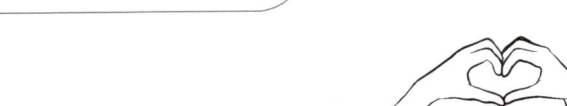

Selfcare Meter
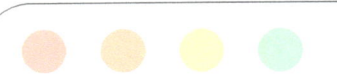

Baby Movement Meter
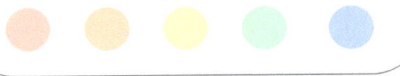

Memorable Moments

_____
_____
_____
_____
_____
_____
_____

Current Concerns

_____
_____
_____
_____
_____
_____

Prep Efforts

_____
_____
_____
_____
_____

Research prenatal vitamin options:

Notes

Week 5

Baby's Size

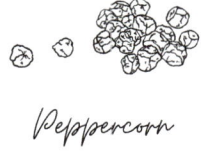

Peppercorn

Major Milestones

- neural tube development continues into spine and brain
- the placenta and umbilical cord grow to support oxygen and nutrient supply to baby

Symptoms

_____
_____
_____
_____
_____
_____
_____
_____

Cravings

_____
_____
_____
_____
_____
_____
_____
_____

Mood Meter

Sleep Meter

Selfcare Meter

Baby Moevement Meter

Memorable Moments

_____
_____
_____
_____
_____
_____
_____

Current Concerns

_____
_____
_____
_____
_____
_____

Prep Efforts

_____
_____
_____
_____
_____
_____

Research birthing and parenting classes in area.

Notes

Week 6

Baby's Size

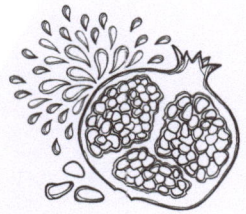

Pomegranate Seed

Major Milestones

- major organ development begins
- pregnancy symptoms including sickness, fatigue, breast tenderness, and mood swings begin

Symptoms

Cravings

Mood Meter

Sleep Meter

Self-care Meter

Baby Moevement Meter

Memorable Moments

_____
_____
_____
_____
_____
_____
_____

Current Concerns

_____
_____
_____
_____
_____

Prep Efforts

_____
_____
_____
_____
_____

Research different birthing options, including locations

Notes:

Week 7

Baby's Size

Blueberry

Major Milestones

- the baby's genitals begin to form
- bones begin to replace soft cartilage, embryo resembles tadpole
- pregnancy cravings begin

Symptoms

Cravings

Mood Meter

Sleep Meter

Selfcare Meter

Baby Moevement Meter

Memorable Moments

_____
_____
_____
_____
_____
_____
_____

Current Concerns

_____
_____
_____
_____
_____
_____

Prep Efforts

_____
_____
_____
_____
_____
_____

Research facilities and services available at potential birthing locations.

Notes

Week 8

Baby's Size

Raspberry

Major Milestones

- toe and finger development begin
- eyes and ears begin to form
- new symptoms, including lower back pain, begins as your uterus continues to grow

Symptoms

Cravings

Mood Meter
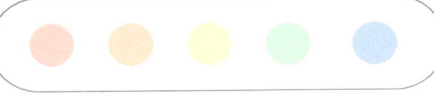

Sleep Meter
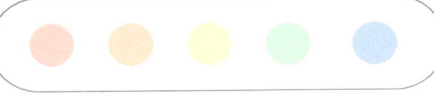

Selfcare Meter
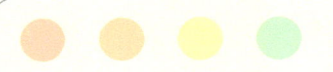

Baby Movement Meter
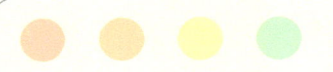

Memorable Moments

_____
_____
_____
_____
_____
_____
_____

Current Concerns

_____
_____
_____
_____
_____
_____

Prep Efforts

_____
_____
_____
_____
_____
_____

Research pain management options.

Notes:

Week 9

Baby's Size

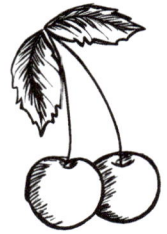

Cherry

Major Milestones
- teeth and taste buds form
- toes and facial features take shape
- morning sickness may begin to fade

Symptoms

Cravings

Mood Meter

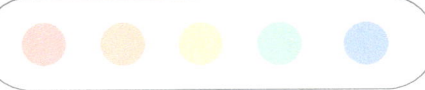

Sleep Meter

Selfcare Meter

Baby Moevement Meter

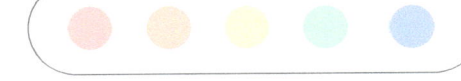

Memorable Moments

_____
_____
_____
_____
_____
_____
_____

Current Concerns

_____
_____
_____
_____
_____
_____

Prep Efforts

_____
_____
_____
_____
_____
_____

Research local childcare options, including programming and cost.

Notes

Week 10

Baby's Size

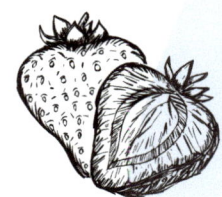

Strawberry

Major Milestones

- arms, legs, feet and toes are fully formed
- nails, external ear, and external genitalia begin to form
- bump may become visible

Symptoms

Cravings

Mood Meter

Sleep Meter

Selfcare Meter

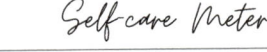

Baby Moevement Meter

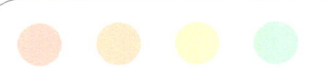

Memorable Moments

_____
_____
_____
_____
_____
_____
_____

Current Concerns

_____
_____
_____
_____
_____
_____

Prep Efforts

_____
_____
_____
_____
_____
_____

Research chestfeeding and nursing options.

Notes

Week 11

Baby's Size

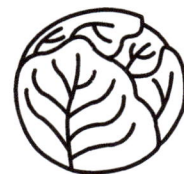

Brussels Sprout

Major Milestones

- baby begins opening hands and mouth
- bones continue hardening and facial features are more prominent
- breast begin to get larger.

Symptoms

Cravings

Mood Meter

Sleep Meter

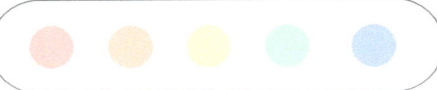

Selfcare Meter

Baby Movement Meter

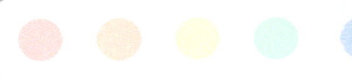

Memorable Moments

_____
_____
_____
_____
_____
_____
_____

Current Concerns

_____
_____
_____
_____
_____
_____

Prep Efforts

_____
_____
_____
_____
_____
_____

Research baby registry options.

Notes

Week 12

Baby's Size

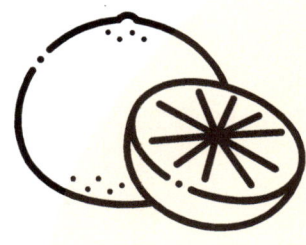

Lime

Major Milestones

- organs, limbs, bones and muscles all fully formed
- circulatory, digestive and urinary systems are working

Symptoms

Cravings

Mood Meter
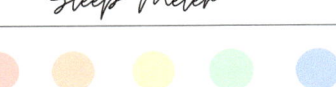

Sleep Meter

Self-care Meter
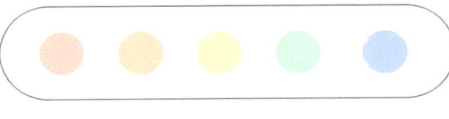

Baby Movement Meter

Memorable Moments

_____
_____
_____
_____
_____
_____
_____

Current Concerns

_____
_____
_____
_____
_____

Prep Efforts

_____
_____
_____
_____
_____

baby gear including crib, car seat, and strollers.

Notes:

1st Trimester Ultrasound

Date

Time

Location

Procedure Performed By

Feelings and Reflection

_____
_____
_____
_____
_____

Things to Rember

-
-

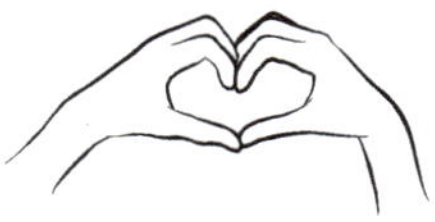

1st Trimester Ultrasound

Date

Time

Location

Procedure Performed By

Feelings and Reflection

_____
_____
_____
_____
_____

Things to Rember

-
-

SECOND TRIMESTER

Week 13

Baby's Size

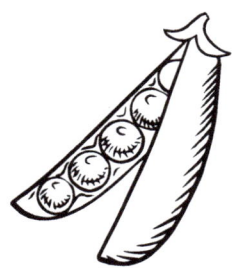

Pea Pod

Major Milestones

- vocal cords form and fetus's head begins to grow proportionate to body
- colostrum may begin leaking from breasts

Symptoms

Cravings

Mood Meter

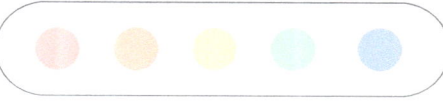

Sleep Meter

Self-care Meter

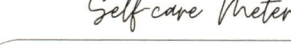

Baby Moevement Meter

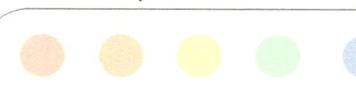

Memorable Moments

_____
_____
_____
_____
_____
_____
_____

Current Concerns

_____
_____
_____
_____
_____

Prep Efforts

_____
_____
_____
_____
_____

Research pediatrician, including experience and approach.

Notes:

Week 14

Baby's Size

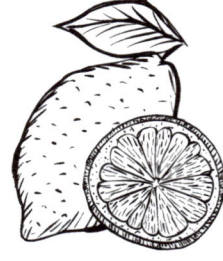

Lemon

Major Milestones

- skin thickens and hair begins to grow
- fingerprints begin forming
- you may experience increased energy

Symptoms

Cravings

Mood Meter

Sleep Meter

Selfcare Meter

Baby Moevement Meter

Memorable Moments

Current Concerns

Prep Efforts

Research nursery themes and designs.

notes

Week 15

Baby's Size

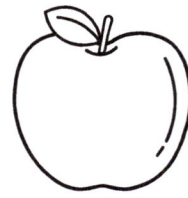

Apple

Major Milestones

- lungs begin to develop
- baby begins to smile and make movements like suck thumb
- increased energy and ease of most symptoms

Symptoms

_____

_____

_____

_____

_____

_____

_____

_____

Cravings

_____

_____

_____

_____

_____

_____

_____

_____

Mood Meter

Sleep Meter

Selfcare Meter

Baby Movement Meter

Memorable Moments

_____
_____
_____
_____
_____
_____
_____
_____

Current Concerns

_____
_____
_____
_____
_____

Prep Efforts

_____
_____
_____
_____
_____

Research baby clothing brands and materials to ensure comfort.

Notes:

Week 16

Baby's Size

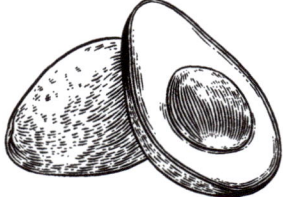

Avocado

Major Milestones

- head is erect
- eyes can slowly move
- skin begins to get thicker

Symptoms

Cravings

Mood Meter
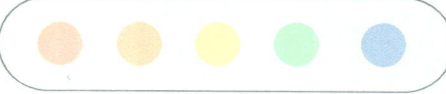

Sleep Meter
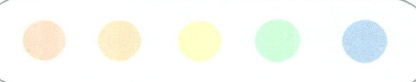

Selfcare Meter
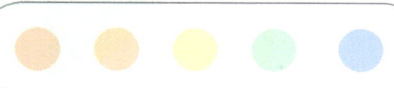

Baby Movement Meter
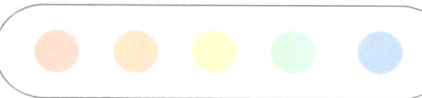

Memorable Moments

Current Concerns

Prep Efforts

Research pospartum care options.

Notes:

Week 17

Baby's Size

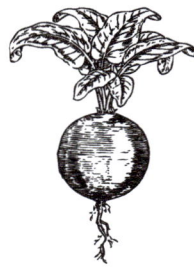

Beet

Major Milestones

- fetus begins to develop fat and skin is covered with vernix, protecting skin from amniotic fluid exposure
- faint belly flutters may begin

Symptoms

Cravings

Mood Meter

Sleep Meter
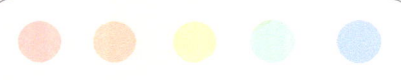

Self-care Meter

Baby Moevement Meter

Memorable Moments

Current Concerns

Prep Efforts

Research baby carriers and slings.

Notes:

Week 18

Baby's Size

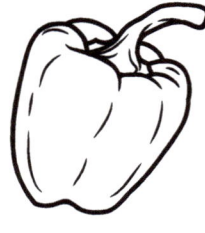

Pepper

Major Milestones

- Bones start to harden
- fetus is covered with hair to provide heat and protection
- baby develops sleep-wake cycle

Symptoms

Cravings

Mood Meter

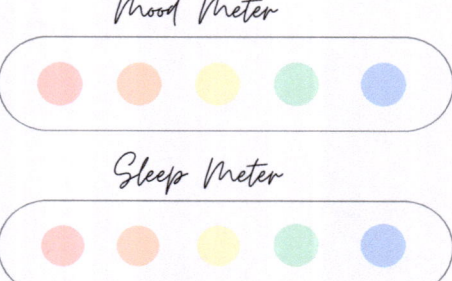

Sleep Meter

Self-care Meter

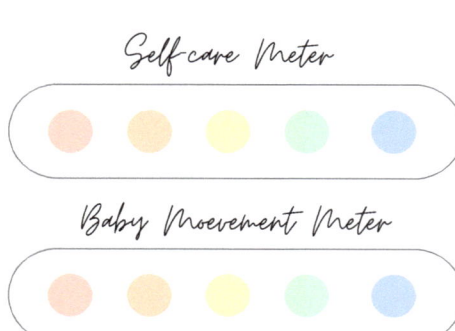

Baby Moevement Meter

Memorable Moments

Current Concerns

Prep Efforts

Research ways to introduce age appropriate foods.

Notes:

Week 19

Baby's Size

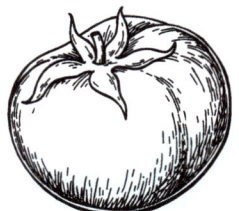

Heirloom Tomato

Major Milestones

- fetus becomes stronger, movement increases
- fetus has fingerprints and can hiccup
- kidneys are formed and begin to function

Symptoms

Cravings

Mood Meter

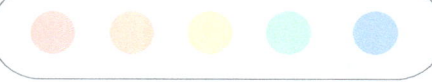

Sleep Meter

Self-care Meter

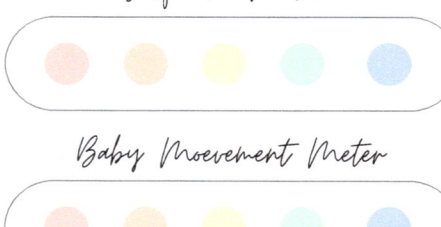

Baby Movement Meter

Memorable Moments

_____
_____
_____
_____
_____
_____
_____

Current Concerns

_____
_____
_____
_____
_____

Prep Efforts

_____
_____
_____
_____
_____

Research types and features of baby monitors.

Notes:

Week 20

Baby's Size

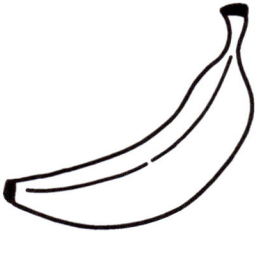

Banana

Major Milestones

- area of brain responsible for senses begins to develop
- nails complete development

Symptoms

Cravings

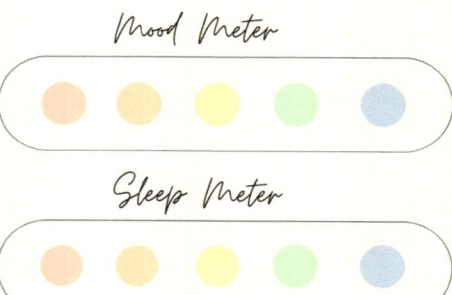

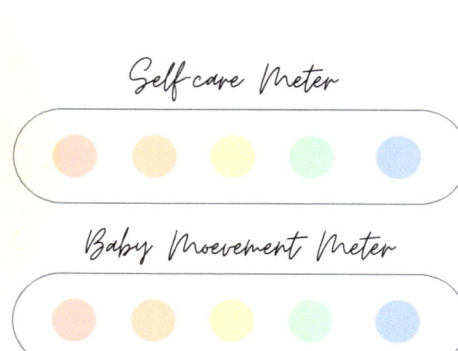

Memorable Moments

_____
_____
_____
_____
_____
_____
_____
_____

Current Concerns

_____
_____
_____
_____
_____
_____

Prep Efforts

_____
_____
_____
_____
_____
_____

Research baby bath products.

Notes

Week 21

Baby's Size

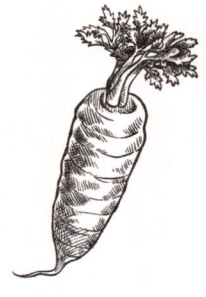

Carrot

Major Milestones

- limb movement is frequent and purposeful
- bone marrow has developed, producing red blood cells

Symptoms

Cravings

Mood Meter

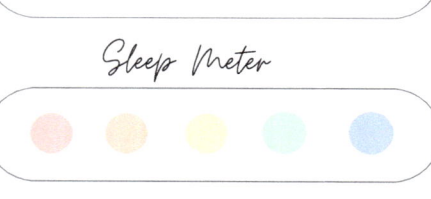

Sleep Meter

Self-care Meter

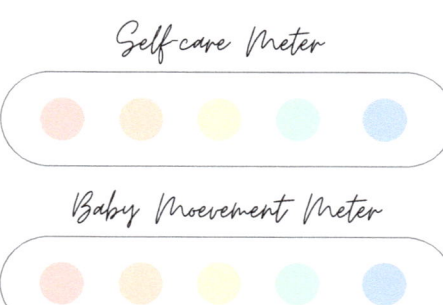

Baby Moevement Meter

Memorable Moments

Current Concerns

Prep Efforts

Research methods for baby-proofing the home.

Notes:

Week 22

Baby's Size

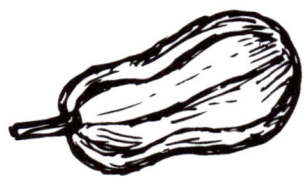

Spaghetti Squash

Major Milestones

- fetus can hear your heartbeat
- tiny eyebrows have formed
- you may begin feeling mild contractions in your abdomen, this is normal

Symptoms

Cravings

Mood Meter

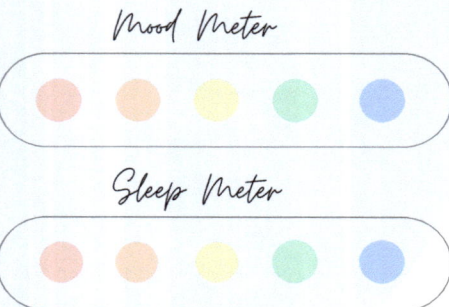

Sleep Meter

Selfcare Meter

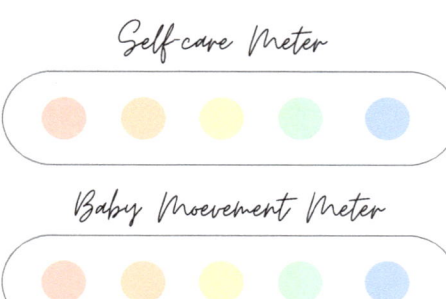

Baby Moevement Meter

Memorable Moments

_____
_____
_____
_____
_____
_____
_____
_____

Current Concerns

_____
_____
_____
_____
_____

Prep Efforts

_____
_____
_____
_____
_____

Research methods for organizing baby supplies.

Notes

Week 23

Baby's Size

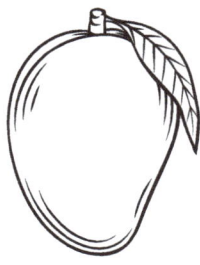

Large Mango

Major Milestones

- fetus is rapidly putting on body fat
- baby may begin responding to your voice

Symptoms

Cravings

Mood Meter

Sleep Meter
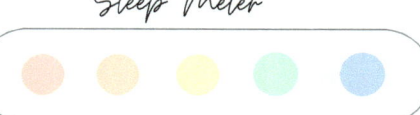

Self-care Meter
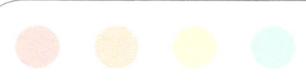

Baby Moevement Meter
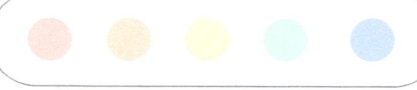

Memorable Moments

_____
_____
_____
_____
_____
_____
_____

Current Concerns

_____
_____
_____
_____
_____

Prep Efforts

_____
_____
_____
_____

Research prenatal exercises and local fitness options.

Notes:

Week 24

Baby's Size

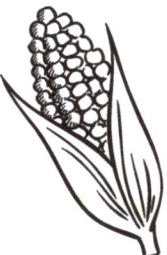

Corn

Major Milestones

- fetus's lungs are fully formed, but not functional outside uterus
- baby bump visibility continues to increase.

Symptoms

Cravings

Mood Meter

Sleep Meter

Selfcare Meter

Baby Moevement Meter

Memorable Moments

_____
_____
_____
_____
_____
_____
_____

Current Concerns

_____
_____
_____
_____
_____

Prep Efforts

_____
_____
_____
_____
_____

Research how to prepare pet for the baby's arrival.

Notes:

Week 25

Baby's Size

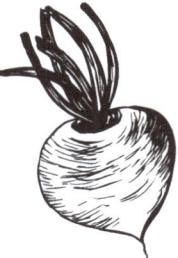

Rutabaga

Major Milestones

- nervous system continues to develop
- fat increase prompts fetus to look less wrinkled

Symptoms

Cravings

Mood Meter

Self-care Meter

Sleep Meter

Baby Moevement Meter

Memorable Moments

_____
_____
_____
_____
_____
_____
_____
_____

Current Concerns

_____
_____
_____
_____
_____

Prep Efforts

_____
_____
_____
_____
_____

Research birthing relaxation strategies.

Notes:

Week 26

Baby's Size

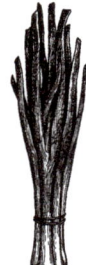

Scallions

Major Milestones

- Fetus makes melanin
- Lungs continue to develop

Symptoms

Cravings

Mood Meter

Sleep Meter

Selfcare Meter

Baby Moevement Meter

Memorable Moments

Current Concerns

Prep Efforts

Research techniques to sooth a newborn.

Notes:

2nd Trimester Ultrasound

Date

Time

Location

Procedure Performed By

Feelings and Reflection

_____
_____
_____
_____
_____

Things to Rember

-
-

2nd Trimester Ultrasound

Date

Time

Location

Procedure Performed By

Feelings and Reflection

_____
_____
_____
_____
_____
_____

Things to Rember

-
-

THIRD TRIMESTER

Week 27

Baby's Size

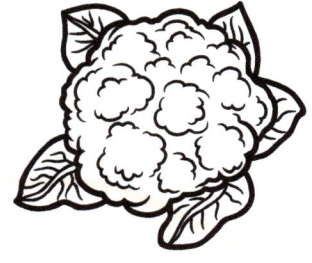

Cauliflower

Major Milestones

- fetus can open eyes and blink
- fetus has eyelashes

Symptoms

_____
_____
_____
_____
_____
_____
_____
_____

Cravings

_____
_____
_____
_____
_____
_____
_____
_____

Mood Meter

Sleep Meter

Self-care Meter

Baby Moevement Meter

Memorable Moments

_____

_____

_____

_____

_____

_____

_____

Current Concerns

_____

_____

_____

_____

_____

Prep Efforts

_____

_____

_____

_____

_____

Research baby carseat safety.

Notes:

Week 28

Baby's Size

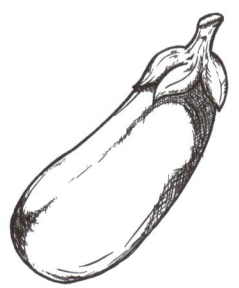

Eggplant

Major Milestones

- fetus begins turning head-down as it prepares for birth

Symptoms

_____
_____
_____
_____
_____
_____
_____

Cravings

_____
_____
_____
_____
_____
_____
_____

Mood Meter

Sleep Meter

Self-care Meter

Baby Movement Meter

Memorable Moments

_____
_____
_____
_____
_____
_____
_____

Current Concerns

_____
_____
_____
_____

Prep Efforts

_____
_____
_____
_____

Research ways to establish a sleep routine.

Notes:

Week 29

Baby's Size

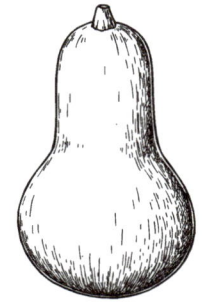

Butternut Squash

Major Milestones

- baby's movements are less intense due to increased amniotic fluid

Symptoms

Cravings

Mood Meter

Sleep Meter

Self-care Meter

Baby Moevement Meter

Memorable Moments

_____
_____
_____
_____
_____
_____
_____

Current Concerns

_____
_____
_____
_____
_____
_____

Prep Efforts

_____
_____
_____
_____
_____
_____

Research ways to introduce your baby to music.

Notes:

Week 30

Baby's Size

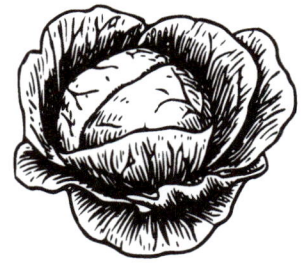

Cabbage

Major Milestones

- fetus can control body heat
- brain is maturing rapidly
- baby begins growing more hair

Symptoms

Cravings

Mood Meter

Sleep Meter

Selfcare Meter

Baby Movement Meter

Memorable Moments

Current Concerns

Prep Efforts

Research ways to introduce your baby to books and literacy.

Notes:

Week 31

Baby's Size

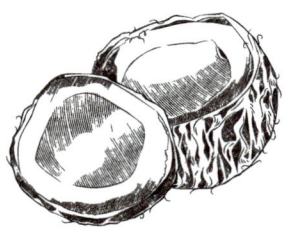

Coconut

Major Milestones

- fetus begins to have distinct sleeping and waking patterns.
- increased bathroom breaks

Symptoms

Cravings

Mood Meter

Sleep Meter

Selfcare Meter

Baby Moevement Meter

Memorable Moments

Current Concerns

Prep Efforts

Research baby gates and safety locks.

Notes

Week 32

Baby's Size

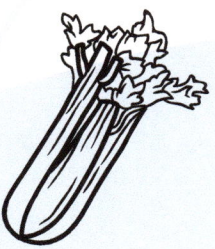

Celery

Major Milestones

- skin, lungs, and brain well-formed

Symptoms

Cravings

Mood Meter

Sleep Meter

Selfcare Meter

Baby Moevement Meter

Memorable Moments

_____

_____

_____

_____

_____

_____

Current Concerns

_____

_____

_____

_____

_____

Prep Efforts

_____

_____

_____

_____

_____

Research postpartum exercises and classes.

Notes:

Week 33

Baby's Size

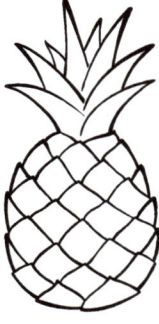

Pineapple

Major Milestones

- bones begin to harden, except for skull to allow passage through birthing canal

Symptoms

Cravings

Mood Meter

Sleep Meter

Self-care Meter

Baby Movement Meter

Memorable Moments

Current Concerns

Prep Efforts

Research early childhood education programs.

Notes:

Week 34

Baby's Size

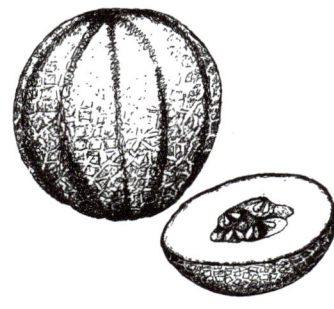
Cantaloupe

Major Milestones

- the vermin, protecting the skin thinking

Symptoms

Cravings

Mood Meter

Sleep Meter

Self-care Meter

Baby Movement Meter

Memorable Moments

Current Concerns

Prep Efforts

Research baby massage and ways to bond with baby.

Notes

Week 35

Baby's Size

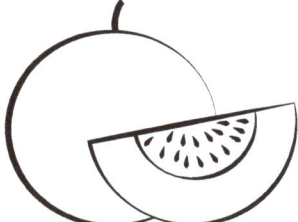

Honeydew Melon

Major Milestones

- brain continues to grow
- circulatory and musculoskeletal systems are fully developed

Symptoms

_____
_____
_____
_____
_____
_____
_____

Cravings

_____
_____
_____
_____
_____
_____
_____

Mood Meter

Sleep Meter

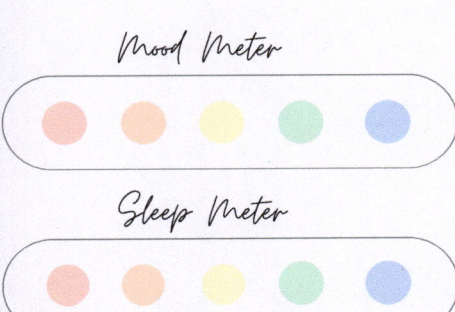

Selfcare Meter

Baby Moevement Meter

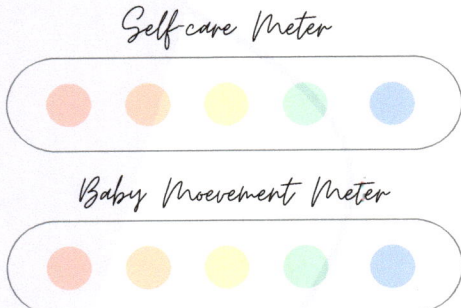

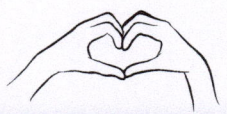

Memorable Moments

Current Concerns

Prep Efforts

Research ways to introduce baby to new sensory situtions.

Notes:

Week 36

Baby's Size

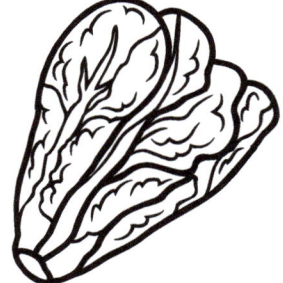

Romaine Lettuce

Major Milestones

- fetus loses its lanugo and wrinkles, looks more like baby you will meet at brith

Symptoms

Cravings

Mood Meter

Sleep Meter

Selfcare Meter

Baby Moevement Meter

Memorable Moments

Current Concerns

Prep Efforts

Research ways to introduce sign language to your baby.

Notes

Week 37

Baby's Size

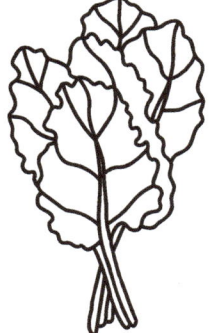

Swiss Chard

Major Milestones

- fetus may begin to drop in pelvis
- begins grasping motions with hands

Symptoms

Cravings

Mood Meter

Sleep Meter

Selfcare Meter

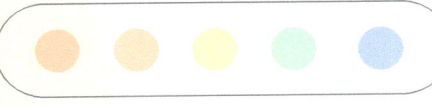

Baby Movement Meter

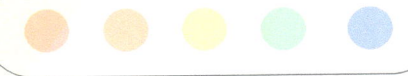

Memorable Moments

Current Concerns

Prep Efforts

Research baby food preperation strategies.

Notes:

Week 38

Baby's Size

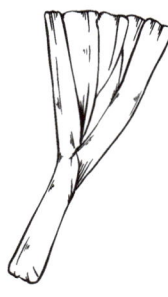

Leeks

Major Milestones

- fetus gains 0.5 pounds per week until birth

Symptoms

Cravings

Mood Meter

Sleep Meter

Selfcare Meter

Baby Moevement Meter

Memorable Moments

Current Concerns

Prep Efforts

Research ways to create a safe outdoor environment.

Notes

Week 39

Baby's Size

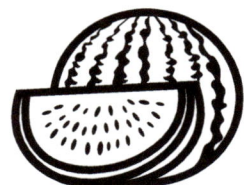

Watermelon

Major Milestones

- fetus is full term

Symptoms

_____
_____
_____
_____
_____
_____
_____
_____

Cravings

_____
_____
_____
_____
_____
_____
_____
_____

Mood Meter

Sleep Meter

Selfcare Meter

Baby Movement Meter

Memorable Moments

Current Concerns

Prep Efforts

Research how to feeding routine and lactation consultants in your area.

Notes

Week 40

Baby's Size

Pumpkin

Major Milestones

- due date, call provider upon signs of labor

Symptoms

_____
_____
_____
_____
_____
_____
_____
_____

Cravings

_____
_____
_____
_____
_____
_____
_____
_____

Mood Meter

Sleep Meter

Selfcare Meter

Baby Moevement Meter

Memorable Moments

Current Concerns

Prep Efforts

Research ways to introduce baby to tummy time.

Notes:

Week 41

Baby's Size

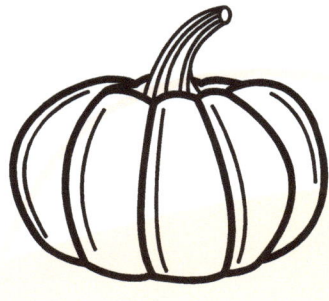

Pumpkin

Major Milestones
- waiting for arrival

Symptoms

Cravings

Mood Meter

Self care Meter

Sleep Meter

Baby Moevement Meter

Week 42

Baby's Size

Pumpkin

Major Milestones
- waiting for arrival

Symptoms

Cravings

Mood Meter

Selfcare Meter

Sleep Meter

Baby Moevement Meter

3rd Trimester Ultrasound

Date

Time

Location

Procedure Performed By

Feelings and Reflection

_____
_____
_____
_____
_____

Things to Rember

-
-

3rd Trimester Ultrasound

Date

Time

Location

Procedure Performed By

Feelings and Reflection

_____
_____
_____
_____
_____

Things to Rember

-
-

FINAL DETAILS

Baby Shower

When | Where | Hosted By

Favorite Games

Favorite Food

Key Memories

_____
_____
_____
_____
_____
_____

Baby Shower

When | Where | Hosted By

Favorite Games

Favorite Food

Key Memories

_____
_____
_____
_____
_____
_____

Baby Names

Name: _____ boy ○ girl ○ neutral ○
Meaning _____

Name: _____ boy ○ girl ○ neutral ○
Meaning _____

Name: _____ boy ○ girl ○ neutral ○
Meaning _____

Name: _____ boy ○ girl ○ neutral ○
Meaning _____

Name: _____ boy ○ girl ○ neutral ○
Meaning _____

Name: _____ boy ○ girl ○ neutral ○
Meaning _____

Name: _____ boy ○ girl ○ neutral ○
Meaning _____

Name: _____ boy ○ girl ○ neutral ○
Meaning _____

Baby Names

name: _____ boy ○ girl ○ neutral ○
meaning _____

name: _____ boy ○ girl ○ neutral ○
meaning _____

name: _____ boy ○ girl ○ neutral ○
meaning _____

name: _____ boy ○ girl ○ neutral ○
meaning _____

name: _____ boy ○ girl ○ neutral ○
meaning _____

name: _____ boy ○ girl ○ neutral ○
meaning _____

name: _____ boy ○ girl ○ neutral ○
meaning _____

Top 3 Names

Birth Plan

Birth Type: Vaginal ○   C-Section ○   Home birth ○

Other: _____

Birthing Parters   Contact Numbers

1. _____
2. _____
3. _____
4. _____

Wishes during delivery...

Birth Environment

Music
_____

Lighting
_____

Scents
_____

Birthing aids
_____

Pain Management
_____

Birth Positions

_____
_____
_____

Fetal Monitoring

_____
_____

Cord Clamping and Cutting

Newborn Care

Bathing

Skin-to-skin contact

Eye Ointment

Other

Breastfeeding or Formula

Postpartum Care

Other

When in labor...

Step 1/ Call Healthcare Provider

Name:_____ Number:_____

Location:_____

🔴🟠🟡🟢🔵🟣🟪

Step 2/ Time Contractions

Time Started:_____ Time of first 1-min contraction:_____

🔴🟠🟡🟢🔵🟣🟪

Step 3/ Gather Essentials

The baby bag should include....

1_____ 1_____
2_____ 10_____
3_____ 11_____
4_____ 12_____
5_____ 13_____
6_____ 14_____
7_____ 15_____
8_____ 16_____

🔴🟠🟡🟢🔵🟣🟪

Step 4/ Use your coping techniques, stay hydrated and nourished, and enjoy every moment of this experience. This is truly once in a LIFETIME!